TaiChi
— handbook —

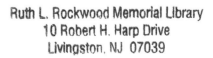

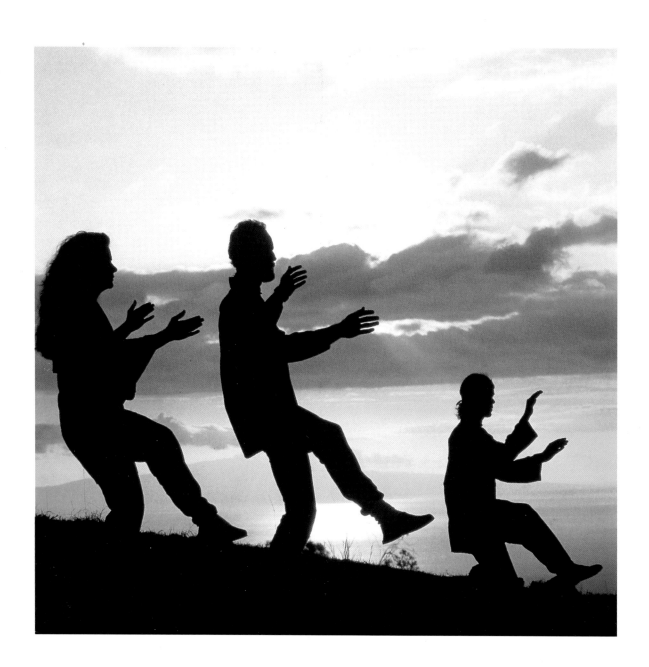

Tai Chi
— handbook —

How to use the ancient art of Tai Chi for health, suppleness and well-being; an easy-to-follow guide with over 200 step-by-step photographs

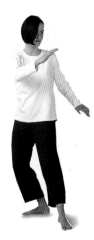

Paul Tucker

Special photography by Don Last

southwater

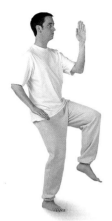

This edition is published by Southwater

Southwater is an imprint of Anness Publishing Ltd
Hermes House, 88–89 Blackfriars Road,
London SE1 8HA
tel. 020 7401 2077; fax 020 7633 9499
www.southwaterbooks.com; info@anness.com

© Anness Publishing Ltd 1997, 2006

Previously published as *Tai Chi*

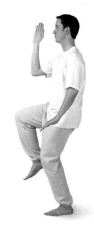

UK agent: The Manning Partnership Ltd, 6 The Old Dairy,
Melcombe Road, Bath BA2 3LR; tel. 01225 478444;
fax 01225 478440;
sales@manning-partnership.co.uk

UK distributor: Grantham Book Services Ltd, Isaac Newton Way,
Alma Park Industrial Estate, Grantham, Lincs NG31 9SD;
tel. 01476 541080; fax 01476 541061; orders@gbs.tbs-ltd.co.uk

North American agent/distributor: National Book Network, 4501
Forbes Boulevard, Suite 200, Lanham, MD 20706;
tel. 301 459 3366; fax 301 429 5746; www.nbnbooks.com

Australian agent/distributor: Pan Macmillan Australia, Level 18,
St Martins Tower, 31 Market St, Sydney, NSW 2000;
tel. 1300 135 113; fax 1300 135 103;
customer.service@macmillan.com.au

New Zealand agent/distributor: David Bateman Ltd,
30 Tarndale Grove, Off Bush Road, Albany, Auckland;
tel. (09) 415 7664; fax (09) 415 8892

Publisher: Joanna Lorenz
Editor: Fiona Eaton
Designer: Allan Mole
Photographer: Don Last

Publisher's note:
The reader should not regard the recommendations, ideas and techniques expressed and described in this book
as substitutes for the advice of a qualified medical practitioner or other qualified professional. Any use to which
the recommendations, ideas and techniques are put is at the reader's sole discretion and risk.

1 3 5 7 9 10 8 6 4 2

CONTENTS

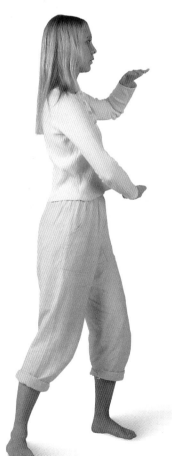

INTRODUCTION

T'ai Chi Ch'uan is an ancient form of slow, graceful and rhythmic exercise which originated in China, where it is still extremely popular, often being performed in public parks in the fresh morning air. It has its roots in Taoist philosophy. The movements of the Tai Chi Form gently tone and strengthen the organs and muscles, improve circulation and posture, and relax both mind and body.

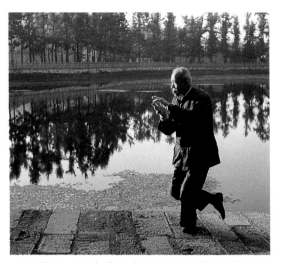

All ages benefit from the gentle art of Tai Chi.

emphasis lies in the yielding aspect of nature overcoming the hard – like the waterfall which eventually wears away the rock beneath. It teaches patience and relaxation, and fosters an understanding of the co-ordination of mind, body and spirit. It is the perfect antidote to the stresses and strains of today's modern lifestyles.

Its name translates as "supreme ultimate fist", but this is not its true meaning. "Strength within softness", "poetry in motion" and "moving harmony" all come closer to expressing the spirit of Tai Chi.

Tai Chi has been variously described as a system of health, medicine, physical co-ordination, relaxation, self-defence and consciousness-raising, as well as a means of exercise and self-development. It is all these things! The style shown in this book is the Yang-style Short Form, as developed by Professor Cheng Man-Ch'ing, which is the most common of the various forms practised in the West.

Unlike the "hard" martial arts which rely on force and speed, Tai Chi is "soft" or "internal". Its

People of all ages, conditions and abilities can benefit from Tai Chi. No special equipment or clothing is needed, and once learned it is with you for the rest of your days – just a little regular practice is all that is needed. The entire Short Form takes only about 12 minutes to complete.

Remember how your body felt when you were a small child: loose, supple, free, full of vitality. As you get older, life's difficulties and traumas – and your responses to them – can add tension upon tension, resulting in stiffness, stress, sickness and fatigue. Tai Chi reconnects your mind and body, helps to relax your joints and muscles, releases tension, gives you a sense of spatial awareness and movement within your environment and increases your understanding of your own and other people's energies.

THE HISTORY OF TAI CHI

Some sources claim Tai Chi is 6000 years old, while more conservative estimates date its beginnings only a few centuries ago. It was traditionally a closely guarded secret passed down through a family. A similar art may have begun in the Tang dynasty (618–906 A.D.), but Chang San-Feng (born 1247) is generally regarded as the founder of Tai Chi, in the Sung dynasty. It is said that as a Taoist monk he saw a crane attacking a snake and was inspired by the soft and yielding nature of the snake, which eventually out-manoeuvred the crane and its hard attacking beak.

Yang Lu-Ch'an (1799–1872) was the founder of Yang style Tai Chi. Legend has it that he learned by spying on Chen Chang-Hsin teaching his students, and was soon able to beat even the advanced ones. Grandmaster Chen was so impressed that he taught Yang all the Chen family Tai Chi skills, reasoning that it was better to spread the essence of Tai Chi to the world than to risk losing its vitality by restricting it to family members only.

Yang Jien-Hou (1839–1917) was the third son of Yang Lu-Ch'an, and also became a famous exponent of Tai Chi. His third son, Yang Cheng-Fu (1883–1936), realized that Tai Chi could improve the health and lift the spirit of the entire nation: he taught Cheng Man-Ch'ing for seven years. The current Yang Forms were defined and regulated by Yang Cheng-Fu, and modified by Cheng Man-Ch'ing (1901–1975), who removed some of the repetition from the Form while retaining its essence.

Following the Cultural Revolution, many great teachers went to South-east Asia, especially Taiwan, Singapore and Malaysia. Cheng Man-Ch'ing took Tai Chi to New York in the mid-1960s and Gerda Geddes introduced it to Britain. Since then it has continued to flourish around the world.

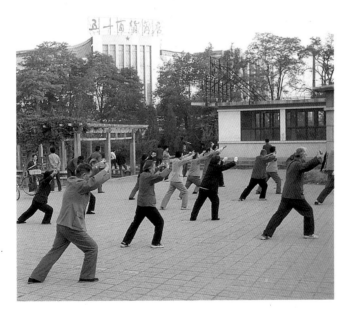

Chinese people practise Tai Chi together in parks in the morning air.

TAI CHI FOR HEALTH OR SELF-DEFENCE?

Although Tai Chi can eventually be used in self-defence, and most classes do incorporate some of its practical applications, it is initially practised mainly for its health-giving benefits. It is particularly useful for increasing alertness and body awareness, and for developing concentration and sensitivity. It helps with balance and posture, and enhances a sense of "groundedness". However, all the postures have a validity in defending yourself against an attack by an opponent. Its gentleness and subtlety do not preclude it being a very effective form of self-defence.

It is not easy to separate the physical and mental aspects of Tai Chi, as they are closely inter-related. In Chinese medicine, the interdependence of mind, body and spirit is seen as integral to well-being. Physical symptoms will affect the emotions and the psyche, and mental troubles will affect your health. In Tai Chi the cat-like alertness required, the relaxed mind, the softening and opening of the joints, the balance and the flow of Chi evenly through the body are all equally important for health and self-defence.

Once you have attained these qualities, which may take many years, you can start to work on increasing the speed in order to practise applications with a partner, while still maintaining the precision, balance and relaxation that are inherent in Tai Chi.

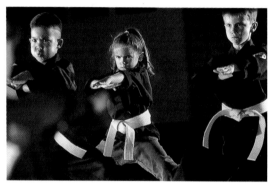

Above: Younger children are encouraged to learn "hard" martial arts such as karate before beginning Tai Chi.
Left: Partner work often incorporates "Sticking Hands".
Facing page: "Pushing Hands".

THE THEORY OF TAI CHI

Like music, Tai Chi cannot be appreciated purely on an intellectual level. It has to be experienced in order to gain an understanding. However, it is useful to look at some of the concepts which are fundamental to the martial arts, as well as to medicine and philosophy. Although treated separately in the West, all these are inseparable in the Eastern view. From thousands of years of close observation of patterns of energy, the Chinese evolved a system of healing that can be used both as preventive medicine and for the treatment of disease.

CHI

Chi is the driving force of human life, the spark behind thought, creativity and growth which maintains and nurtures us. It can be felt as movement of energy in the body, like the flow of an electrical current.

Chi flows through the body along channels called meridians, as blood flows along arteries and veins. When there is a blockage, Chi cannot flow adequately to nourish the organs, and illness results. The concept of Chi is at the very centre of Tai Chi, which aims to restore balance so that Chi flows freely.

THE TAN TIEN

The Chi is stored in the Tan Tien. This is an area about the size of a golf ball, located four finger-widths below the navel, and about one-third of the way from the front to the back of the body. It is the centre of gravity of the body, and in Tai Chi all movement emanates from it. Try to let the breath and the mind sink to the Tan Tien.

YIN AND YANG

Yin and Yang describe the complementary yet opposing forces of nature, such as night and day, cold and hot, female and male, winter and summer, death and life.

Their relationship has a harmony and balance: both Yin and Yang are necessary, they are constantly moving and balancing each other, and the interaction between them creates Chi. The Chinese observed that when the balance of Yin and Yang is disrupted in an individual, so too will be the body's Chi, leading to ill health.

9

FINDING A CLASS

Tai Chi cannot be learned from a book alone (or even a video), and it's important to find a class that you feel comfortable in. You may prefer the intensity of learning with a very small group, or you may enjoy the energy created by a large one. It is important to have good sight lines in order to be able to see the teacher's movements, and sufficient space around you.

One of the joys of Tai Chi is that no special equipment or clothing is needed, simply a small area, well ventilated and with good natural light. Practise outdoors if you can, but most students are apprehensive at first and don't like to feel exposed to the elements – and curious onlookers.

Wear loose, comfortable clothing and flat-soled shoes (not trainers or sneakers), although Tai Chi can be performed in bare or stockinged feet.

The emphasis is on small amounts of regular practice, preferably a few minutes each day. Normally a new "posture" will be learned each week. Repetition and correction of the postures in class is important. Some of the adjustments made may feel only very minor, but they will be significant in allowing the Chi to circulate around the body more freely.

The scope for refining and improving your Tai Chi is limitless. Some of the great masters now in their 70s and 80s have been practising daily since they were children. Each of us needs to find our own level of practice and commitment, but one thing is certain: it cannot be hurried.

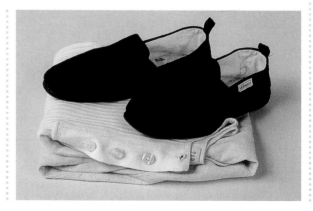

Above: Finding a good class is essential for your progress.
Below: Tai Chi slippers can be worn.

THE PRINCIPLES OF TAI CHI

When you begin you may feel awkward and clumsy. Beginners are often surprised at their lack of co-ordination and balance, and at the differences in mobility between their right and left sides. If you have tended to lean slightly to your left for years, when you straighten up it will feel as though you are tilted to the right. This may take a while to change. As you learn to relax and feel more comfortable with a new way of moving, the positions and steps start to feel more natural. Be patient and diligent: perfecting the moves can take a lifetime.

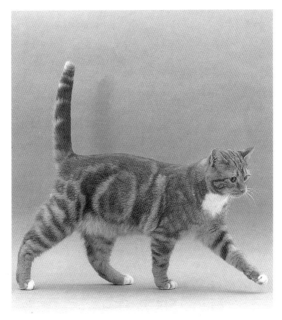

Tai Chi movements have been likened to a cat taking a tentative step as it walks.

upper body should feel light and agile, free and flexible. Your lower body should feel heavy and well grounded.

• Establish a solid "root" with the ground – imagine small roots growing from the soles of your feet into the earth.

• Align the joints of your shoulder, hip, knee and ankle vertically, so that gravity keeps your body in alignment rather than muscular effort. Never lock any of the joints.

• Let your tongue rest lightly on the roof of your mouth.

• Let your mind begin the movement, which comes up through the legs, is directed by the waist and flows out through the fingertips.

• Relax. This is the basic principle. The body needs to be loose and open so that Chi can flow freely. Allow tension to sink from your upper body down through your legs to the soles of your feet and into the earth.

• Allow your mind and your Chi to settle into the Tan Tien. Sinking your chest slightly helps this to happen. Relax your shoulders and elbows. Your

• Be in the present moment, focusing on what is actually happening, not thinking about the move just past or the one to come.

• Never use force. Avoid wasting energy. Let your movements be light, nimble and effortless.

• Seek stillness within movement. Seek serenity within activity.

WARM-UP EXERCISES

Perform these exercises slowly and gently, with the mind and the breath focused in the Tan Tien. Notice any differences between the right and left sides of your body, and between the upper and lower parts. Be aware of the harmonious interrelationships of all the various parts of your body as you move and breathe. Concentrate, too, on the natural expansion and contraction of your lungs, and the movement of your ribcage at the sides and back of your body as well as at the front.

All the exercises in this chapter are performed with the feet shoulder-width apart and parallel to each other unless otherwise stated. However, for those unable to stand, most of the exercises can also be done in a sitting position and great benefit can still be obtained from them.

EXERCISE 1
Circling Hands

This is a very calming exercise which may be repeated for several minutes.

1 Inhale and allow both hands to float upwards a comfortable distance in front of your body, palms facing downwards.

2 As your hands rise above your head, relax the wrists and begin to open the palms outwards.

3 As you exhale, continue to open out your arms to your sides, palms facing upwards. Draw your hands inwards at the bottom of the circle, ready to turn over and begin a new circle.

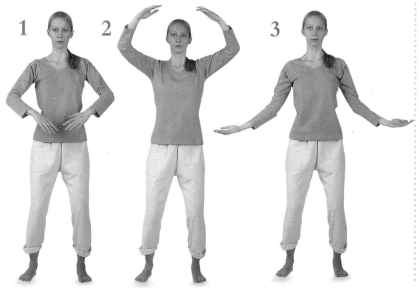

EXERCISE 2
Push to Heaven and Earth

Throughout this exercise, there is a changing relationship between the hands, whether they are facing towards or away from each other. Co-ordinate your breathing so that as the breath changes from inhalation to exhalation, or vice versa, so the hands change their direction.

1 Breathe in and let both hands float up in front of your body, palms upwards. As you exhale, your right hand pushes down towards earth, ending up by your right hip, while your left hand turns over and pushes up towards heaven, finishing above your left temple. Feel a diagonal stretch through your entire body.

2 Breathe in again, relaxing your palms which now turn to face each other and begin moving towards each other in front of your body. Feel as if there is a ball of energy between your hands.

3 Turn your right palm over and outwards as you exhale. Continue to push your right hand upwards until it arrives above your right temple, while your left hand now pushes down, finishing by your left hip.

4 Breathe in again and bring your hands in front of your body in a mirror image of Step 2.

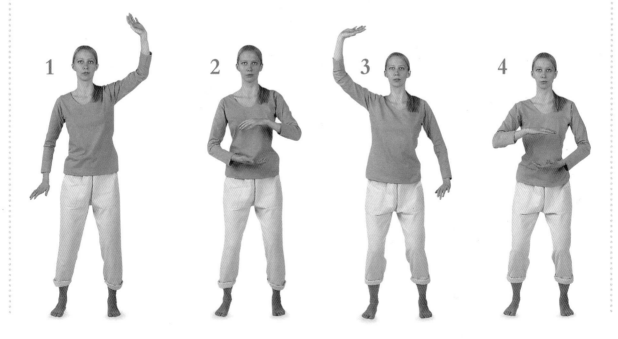

EXERCISE 3
Shaking out Shoulders, Arms and Hands

▶ Gently shake out any tension in your wrists and hands. Gradually work up to include your shoulders. This exercise is especially useful before, during and after long periods at a keyboard, or for anyone who does intricate or repetitive work with the hands.

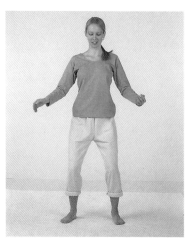

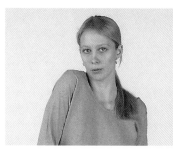

EXERCISE 4
Loosening Shoulders

◀ Make increasing circles with one shoulder. Change direction and decrease the size of the circles. Repeat for the other shoulder. Rotate your shoulders alternately.

EXERCISE 5
Loosening Wrists

▶ Ensure that each finger is lightly touching the thumb. The feeling should be one of holding a droplet of water. Make circles with your hands, keeping your arms and shoulders relaxed.

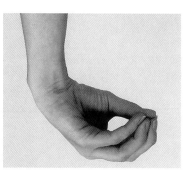

EXERCISE 6
Rotating Waist

▽ Place both hands lightly on your hips. Keeping your head up, begin by spiralling your hips slowly outwards, feeling for any restriction, tightness or lack of ease. Change direction and spiral back in slowly.

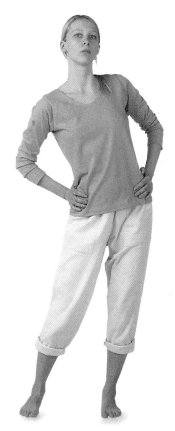

14

EXERCISE 7
Knee Rotations

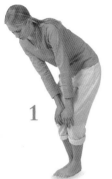

1 Bring your feet together and place your palms lightly on your upper kneecaps. Feel the Chi from your palms radiating deep into your knee joints. Circle your knees clockwise several times, then change direction.

2 Keep your legs and hands in the same position. Rotate your knees in opposite directions – one circles clockwise while the other circles anti-clockwise (counter-clockwise). Change the direction of each knee and repeat the rotations.

EXERCISE 9
Calf Stretch

◀ Turn out your left foot to 45° and step forward with your right foot. Keeping the heel on the floor, pull up your toes towards the knee. Drop your body forward, keeping your right leg straight and letting your hands hang down. Hold for a few breaths and release. Repeat for the other leg.

EXERCISE 8
Shaking Out Legs and Feet

▼ Stand on one leg while gently shaking tension from the other leg for 10–15 seconds. Repeat for the other leg.

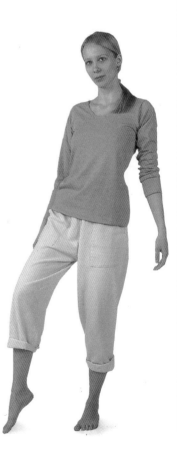

EXERCISE 10
Four-directional Breathing

1 As you inhale, bring your hands up to chest height, palms facing upwards.

2 As you exhale, turn the palms to face away and extend your arms as if pushing something away.

3 On the next inhalation, turn your palms back to face your body, softening your arms and drawing them back in towards your chest.

4 Exhale again, turn the palms out and extend your arms out to your sides.

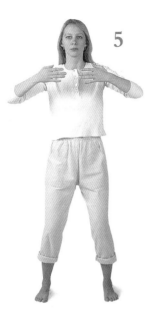

5

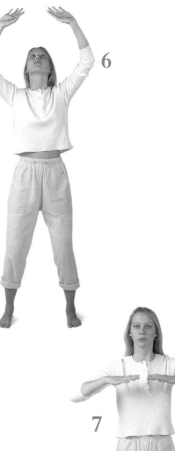

6

5 Relax and bring your arms in towards your chest as you inhale.

6 On the next exhalation turn your palms upwards and extend your arms towards the sky.

7 Breathe in again and let your arms descend, palms facing downwards.

8 As your arms and hands pass the Tan Tien, begin breathing out and pushing down towards the earth. On the next inhalation the hands come up and a new cycle of four breaths begins. Repeat this sequence several times.

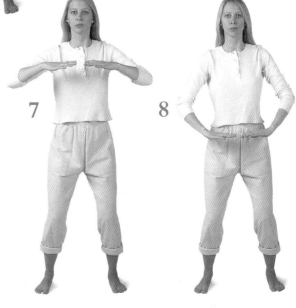

7

8

EXERCISE 11
Rotating from the Waist with Feet Forward

1 Imagine a central axis from the crown of your head, dropping down through your body to a point between your feet. Rotate your body around this axis, keeping your arms relaxed. Try to keep each knee over its respective big toe, and shift your weight from one leg to the other as you turn.

2 As your waist turns to the left, your weight shifts on to your left leg. As it turns right, move your weight across on to your right leg. Let your arms swing naturally, following the movement of your waist. Repeat the sequence for about 1 minute.

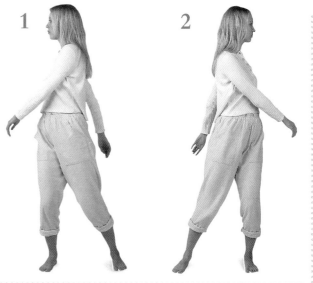

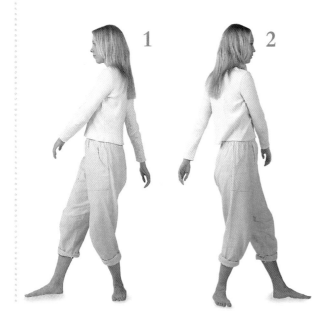

EXERCISE 12
Rotating from the Waist with Feet Pivoting on the Heel

This is similar to the previous exercise, but the weight shifts differently.

1 Bring all your weight on to your left leg and turn your waist to the right, simultaneously turning your right foot out to 90°.

2 As your waist returns to the centre, the right toes come around. The right heel remains on the ground. Then, as you turn your waist to the left, transfer your weight completely to your right leg and pivot on your left heel, turning the toes through 90°. Gradually increase the speed until you find a comfortable, gentle rhythm. Continue for about 1 minute.

EXERCISE 13
Rotating from the Waist Turning on the Ball of the Foot

In this exercise, the movement of the waist is exactly as in the previous two exercises. The arms also follow the same movement, but each foot pivots in turn on the ball.

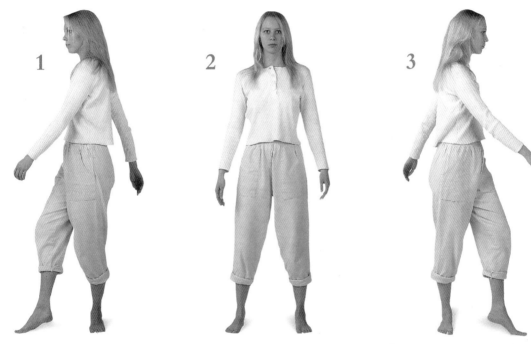

1 Keeping your weight in your left leg, turn your waist to the right. Lift your right heel and swivel the right foot through 90°.

2 As your waist returns to the centre, straighten your right foot until your feet are parallel and shoulder-width apart. Transfer your weight on to your right foot.

3 Turn your waist to the left, lift your left heel and pivot on the ball of your left foot. Turn back to the centre and repeat the sequence for about 1 minute, keeping your head up, back straight and arms and shoulders relaxed.

EXERCISE 14
Opening and Closing the Circle

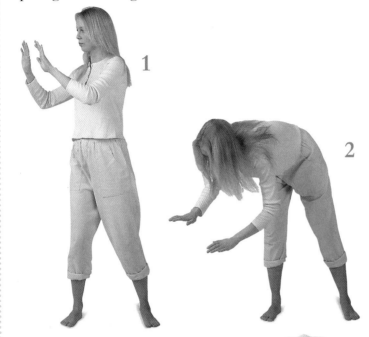

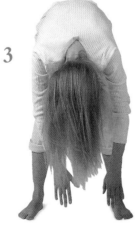

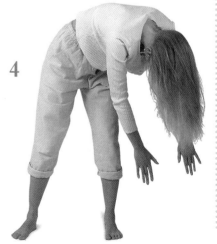

1 Place your hands in front of your face, palms facing away. Turn your waist slowly to the right.

2 Drop your weight into your right leg and continue turning your waist, which in turn brings your hands around in a large circular movement.

3 As your hands cross the bottom of the circle, shift your weight into your left leg.

4 Continue to turn your waist slowly, bringing your hands up to complete the circle.

20

5 When your hands reach their starting-point in front of your face, repeat the sequence and continue for several more rotations.

6 Change direction gently at the bottom of the circle to repeat the sequence. This time, join your palms together lightly at the top of each circle.

7 Keep the palms together as you turn, allowing your hands to separate at the bottom of the circle. Remember to move from the waist and transfer your weight.

8 Finish the exercise by keeping your palms connected and spiralling your hands in slowly to end in front of your chest.

EXERCISE 15
Arm Rotations

1 Turn out your right foot to 45° and take a shoulder-width step forwards with your left foot. Bring 70% of your weight on to your left leg, and rest your left hand on your hip. Form a loose fist with your right hand and rotate the arm backwards three times, then forwards three times in a large circle. Repeat twice.

2 Turn out your left foot to 45° and take a shoulder-width step forwards with your right foot. Bring 70% of your weight on to your right leg, and rest your right hand on your hip, in a mirror image of Step 1. Form a loose fist with your left hand and rotate the arm backwards three times, then forwards three times in a large circle. Repeat twice.

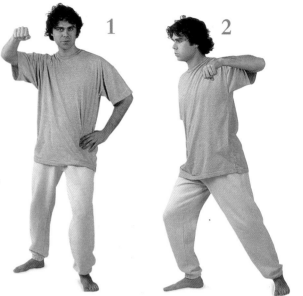

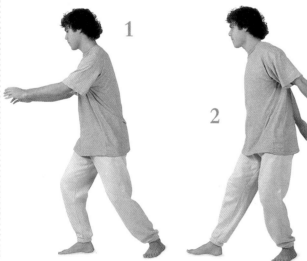

EXERCISE 16
Shifting Weight

1 Place your left foot at 45° and your right foot pointing forward, with heels shoulder-width apart. Shift your weight from one leg to the other, keeping the Tan Tien on a horizontal plane – do not tip your pelvis forwards or backwards.

2 Let your arms swing naturally with the momentum of the weight shifting. Continue for about 1 minute, then place your right foot at 45° with your left foot forward and repeat. Feel a strong root developing through your feet into the earth.

EXERCISE 17
Stepping Forward, Stepping Back

1 Place your left foot at 45°, right foot pointing forward. Shift all your weight from the left foot to the right, then back on to the left. With no weight on the right foot, pick it up and take a step backwards, toe first.

2 Transfer your weight to the right foot, then back to the left. Take a step forwards with the "empty" right foot, heel first. Repeat this sequence several times, concentrating on the steps being empty of any weight. Repeat the exercise, keeping the right foot rooted to the ground, and stepping with the left foot.

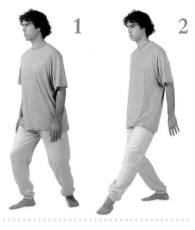

EXERCISE 18
Waving Hands in Clouds

1 Begin with your right hand facing the Tan Tien, your left hand directly above it, facing your chest. Slowly turn your waist to the left, shifting your weight into your left leg. At the same time turn your palms towards each other, as if holding a large ball.

2 Bring your waist back to the front. As you do so, lower your left hand until it is opposite the Tan Tien and raise your right hand to the level of your chest, with your palms facing your body.

3 Now turn your waist to the right, shift the weight across to your right leg, and turn your palms towards each other in a mirror image of Step 1. Repeat the entire sequence several times.

EXERCISE 19 *Push to Centre, Push to Corner*

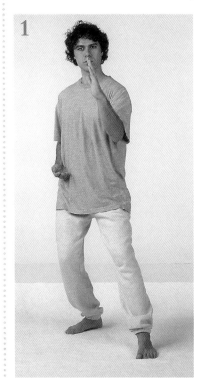

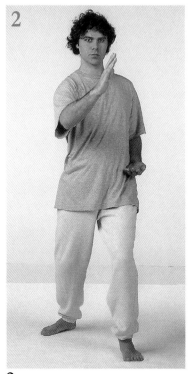

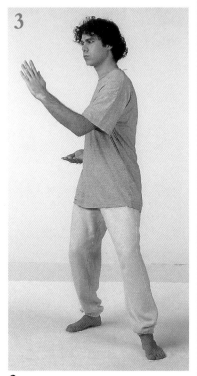

1 Place your right foot at 45° and step forward with your left foot. Begin with all your weight on your right leg, right hand resting palm upwards on your right hip, left fingertips in line with your mouth, palm facing diagonally forwards and to the centre.

2 Bring your weight forward on to your left leg. Your right hand turns diagonally forwards as it comes to push towards the centre of your body; your left hand turns palm upwards as it draws back to rest on your left hip.

3 Shift your weight back on to your right foot, turning your waist 45° to the right. At the same time draw your right hand back to your right hip and push your left hand towards the corner until it is in line with the centre of your body, fingertips opposite your mouth. Repeat Steps 2 and 3 for about 1 minute.

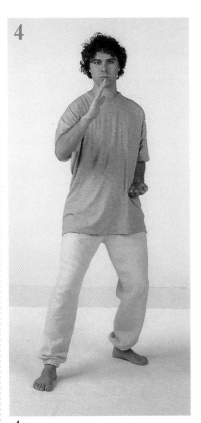

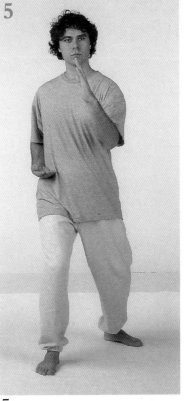

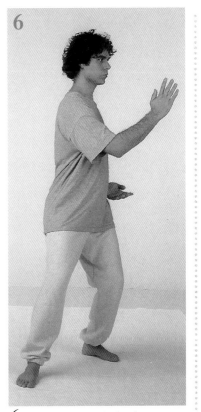

4 Repeat the sequence in mirror image. Place your left foot at 45° and step forward with the right. Begin with all your weight on your left leg, left hand resting palm upwards on your left hip, right fingertips in line with your mouth, palm facing diagonally forwards and to the centre.

5 Bring your weight forward on to your right leg. Your left hand turns diagonally forwards as it comes to push towards the centre of the body, your right hand turns palm upwards as it draws back to rest on the right hip.

6 Shift your weight back on to your left foot, turning your waist through 45° to the left. At the same time, draw your left hand back to your left hip and push your right hand towards the corner until it is in line with the centre of your body, fingertips opposite your mouth. Repeat the cycle in Steps 5 and 6 for about 1 minute.

EXERCISE 20
Rotating Whole Body, Arms in Front

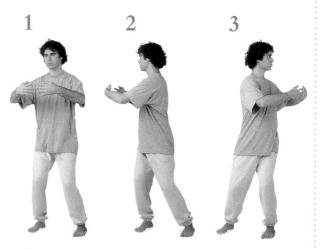

1 Hold both arms horizontally in front of the chest, palms facing inwards, fingertips almost touching. You should feel as if you are holding a large ball, or "hugging a tree".

2 Turn your waist to the right, simultaneously shifting your weight across to your right leg.

3 Return to the centre, then turn to the left and move your weight on to your left leg. Move your arms with the rest of your body each time.

EXERCISE 21
Neck Rotations

▶ Keep the palms of your hands in front of and facing your chest, fingertips almost touching. Relax your shoulders and elbows. Turn your head to look first over one shoulder, then back to the centre before turning to look over the other. Repeat several times, keeping the neck movements as fluid as possible.

EXERCISE 22
Hip Rotations

▶ Turn out your left foot at 45° and sink all your weight on to it. Draw a smooth circle with your right knee, keeping the hip movement as fluid as possible. Repeat the same rotation on the other hip.

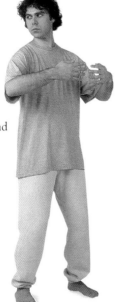

EXERCISE 23 *Ankle Rotations*

As you do this exercise, notice the difference between the right and left ankles – it's surprising to discover that there's often a considerable distinction!

▶ Place your left foot at 45°, bend your left knee and sink all your weight into your left leg. Lift your right foot and slowly rotate the ankle, describing a circle with your big toe. Repeat the exercise for the left ankle.

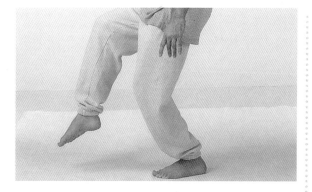

EXERCISE 24 *Return to Centre*

This exercise is the reverse of Exercise 1, "Circling Hands".

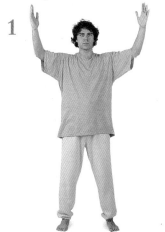
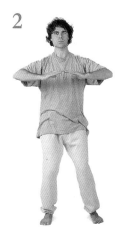
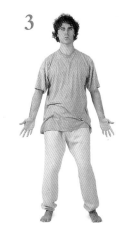

1 As you breathe in, take your hands out to the sides in front of your body, and raise them slowly in a large circle, palms facing upwards.

2 As you exhale, lower your hands in front of the centre of your body, palms facing downwards.

3 At the bottom of the circle, turn your hands outwards again to begin a new circle with the new breath.

EXERCISE 25
Stimulating the Back of the Neck

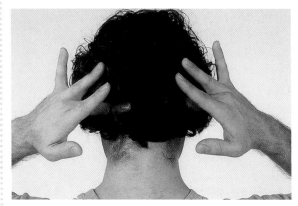

▲ Bring your heels together and turn your feet out, making a right angle at the heels. Lift your hands to the back of your head. Flick your index and middle fingers over each other to tap the base of the occipital ridge at the back of the skull, releasing Chi up to the top of your head. Flick the back of your head about 20 times.

EXERCISE 26
Kidney Massage

The kidneys are the most important organs, according to Chinese medicine, as they store the Chi, so it is important to look after them. This massage provides gentle stimulation and helps to break down crystals of uric acid, a common component of kidney stones.

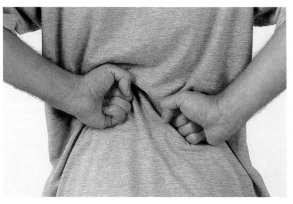

▲ Bring your heels together, as in the previous exercise. Massage around your kidneys with loose fists.

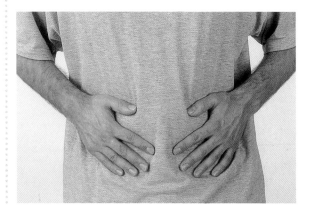

EXERCISE 27
Abdominal Massage

◀ With your heels together, massage your abdomen in a circular motion with the palms of your hands.

EXERCISE 28 *Feeling the Air*

1 With your heels together, inhale and let both hands float up towards your shoulders, palms facing upwards. Feel the resistance of the air on your palms.

2 As you exhale, let both hands float back down. Try to feel resistance on the backs of your hands, and the air rushing softly between your fingers.

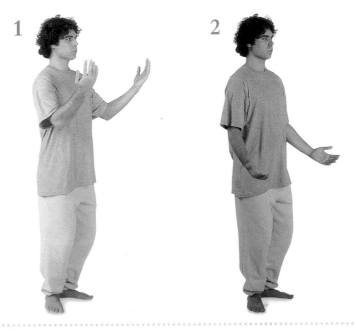

EXERCISE 29
Stillness Within Movement

▶ Bring your heels together at right angles to each other. Try to feel where your body weight naturally lies. Does it tend to be greater on the left or the right foot? Is it nearer the toes or the heel? On the instep or the outer edge of the foot? Is it moving around or still? If moving, is it spiralling, circling or wandering about? Are the movements random or even, chaotic or rhythmical?

You are seeking a point of equilibrium, where you can feel relaxed, still and evenly balanced. Try to let go of any little muscular contractions and other activity. Let the weight settle gently and rest. Just let yourself be quiet and motionless. After a few quiet moments of standing still, you can begin some Tai Chi walking, or start the Form. Notice the feelings you have, especially in the Tan Tien, and carry these feelings with you into the Form.

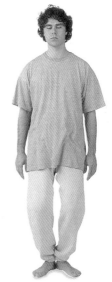

YANG-STYLE SHORT FORM

After completing the warm-up exercises, and a moment or so quietly standing to see if you can find a point of equilibrium, a few minutes of Tai Chi walking may follow. This is walking with an "empty step", rather in the manner of a cat tentatively putting out its paw before committing its full weight to the front leg.

As you progress through the Form, use the following pages as an aide-mémoire for your practice, especially for the transitions from one posture to the next. Remember to keep your movements slow and smooth, like clouds drifting gently by on a summer's day, and - above all - relax!

LESSON 1
Attention, Preparation and Beginning

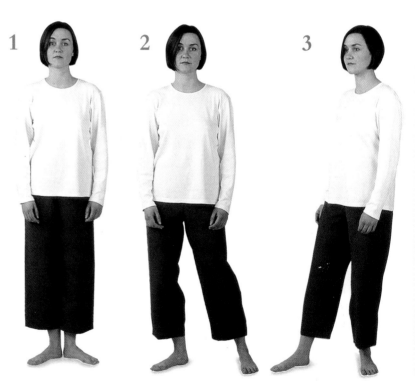

1 Stand in a relaxed and upright posture, feet pointing diagonally outwards, making a right angle. Distribute your weight evenly.

2 Bend your right knee and sink all your weight down through your right leg into the foot, without leaning across. Move the "empty" left leg a shoulder-width away, with the toes pointing straight ahead.

3 Transfer 70% of your weight to your left leg, simultaneously turning your waist (and therefore your whole body) diagonally to the right.

4 Keeping 70% of your weight in your left leg, turn your whole body back to face the front. Bring your right foot around to the front as your waist moves. Your feet should be shoulder-width apart and parallel. Your hands also move with your body, the palms facing the ground as if resting on a cushion of air, just in front of and just below your waist.

5 Relax your wrists and let your arms float up and away from your body. When your hands reach shoulder height, gently extend the fingertips.

6 Draw your hands back in towards your body by dropping the elbows.

7 Relax your wrists and let your hands float down the front of your body, back to where they started, just in front of and just below your waist. The posture ends with another 10% of your weight sunk into your left leg, so that 80% is now in the left and 20% in the right.

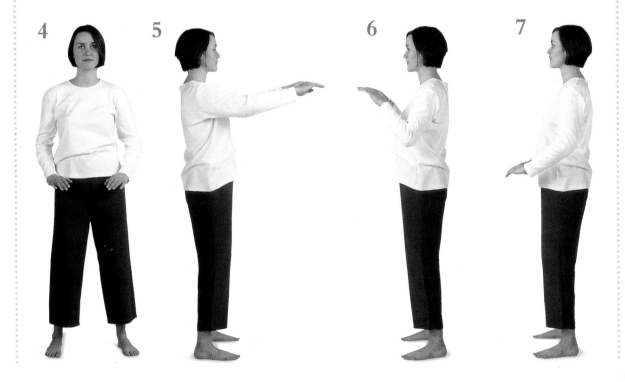

LESSON 2
Ward Off Left

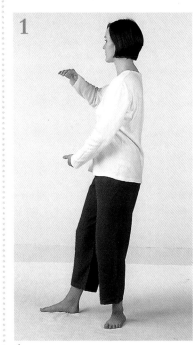

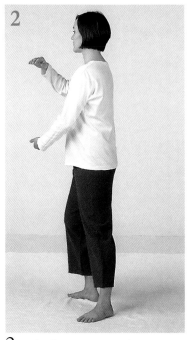

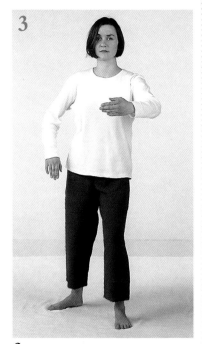

1 Sink all your weight into your left leg. Turn your whole body 90° to the right, pivoting on the empty right heel. There is a feeling of holding a large ball, with the right hand in front of the chest, palm facing down, and the left hand directly under it, palm upwards.

2 Sink all your weight on to your right leg, as if carrying the ball forward. Pick up your empty left leg and step directly forward, toes pointing to the front.

3 Turn your waist to the left, to face the front. As you do so, your left hand comes up, palm facing your chest, and your right hand floats down to just outside your right thigh, palm facing down. Shift 70% of your weight into your left leg, as your right foot simultaneously comes around to 45°. If you were to draw your left foot back, your heels would be shoulder-width apart.

LESSON 3
Ward Off Right

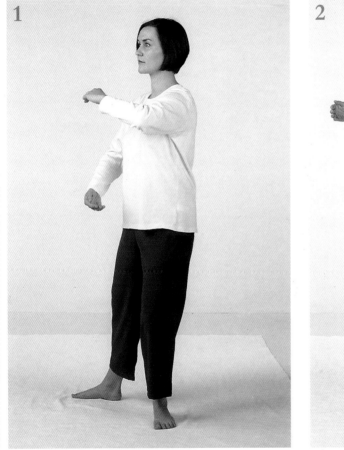

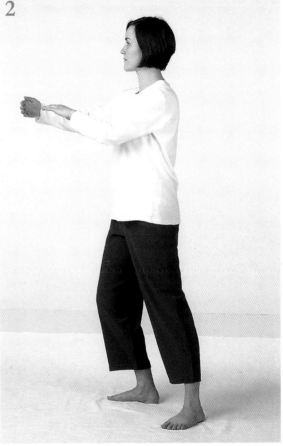

1 Sink all your weight into your left leg. Turn to the right: the left palm turns face down, the right palm turns upwards as if both hands are again holding the large ball. Pick up your right foot and step so that your heels are once more shoulder-width apart.

2 As you turn your waist to face the right-hand side, shift 70% of your weight on to your right foot, and turn your left foot to 45°. Raise your right arm so that the palm faces your chest, the fingertips of your left hand looking into the right palm.

LESSON 4
Roll Back, Press and Push
This posture, together with the one that follows it, "Single Whip", is also known as "Grasping the Sparrow's Tail".

1 Turn your body to the right. Point the fingertips of your right hand to the sky in a relaxed way. Your left arm moves horizontally with the fingertips almost touching the right elbow, palm facing the body. Your weight remains 70% on the right leg, 30% on the left.

2 As you turn your waist to the left, begin to shift weight on to your left leg. Follow the movement of the body with your arms until your right hand is horizontal. Your left hand then begins to flow down with the movement of your waist to the left. Allow all your weight to settle into your left leg.

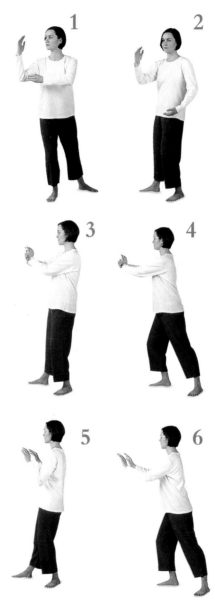

3 Turn your waist back to the right and let your left arm follow this movement. All your weight remains in the left leg. Bring your palm across to rest against your right wrist, opposite the centre of your chest.

4 Press forward, keeping the hands in full contact. Shift 70% of your weight into your front (right) leg. Ensure that your heels are still shoulder-width apart, the right foot pointing forward, the left foot at 45°.

5 Separate your hands and sink all your weight back into your left foot. Your fingertips are now shoulder-width apart at shoulder height.

6 Move your weight forward 70% into your right leg. Your arms and hands keep the same position.

LESSON 5
Single Whip

1 As your weight shifts back into the left leg, leave your fingers where they are in space, effectively straightening – but not locking – your arms. The palms now face the ground.

2 Turn your whole body to the left and shift all your weight into your left leg. Your right heel remains on the ground while your toes turn through 120°, following the body round. Your arms remain parallel at shoulder height and shoulder-width apart.

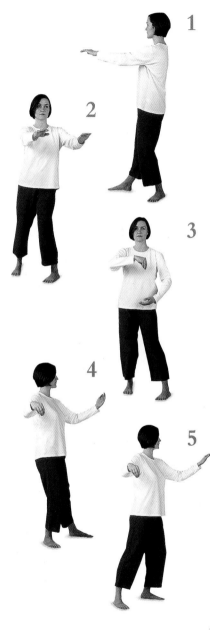

3 Sink your weight back into your right leg. Bring your left hand under the right to hold the imaginary ball in front of your body. Meanwhile, form a "hook" with the fingers and thumb of your right hand, with the thumb connected to each finger as if holding a single droplet of water. The hook of the right hand is directly over the upturned palm of the left hand.

4 Ensure all your weight is in your right leg. Bend the right knee and turn your body to the left, sending out the hook in line with, and at the same height as, your shoulder. Take an empty shoulder-width step with your left foot, the heel connecting with the ground first. The left arm pivots at the elbow.

5 Shift 70% of your weight on to your left leg, adjusting your right foot to 45°. Ensure that your heels are shoulder-width apart, your left hand in line with your left shoulder and your right hand's hook at 90° to the rest of your body.

LESSON 6
Lifting Hands. Shoulder Stroke

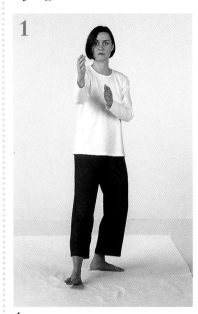

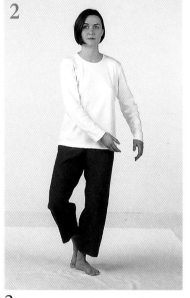

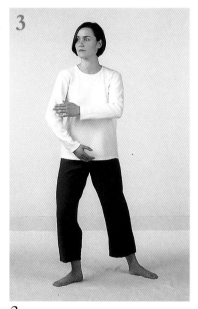

1 Place all your weight on your left leg. Turn your waist to the right. Open your hands and turn the palms inwards, the left palm towards the right elbow. Pick up your empty right foot and place the heel down without weight, in such a position that if you drew the right foot back in a straight line, you would avoid clipping the left heel.

2 Turn your waist to the left, your hands following the movement of your waist. Bring your right toe by your left heel, touching the ground but weightless.

3 Take an empty shoulder-width step to the right with your right foot, heel first. Transfer 70% of your weight forwards into the right foot. Your left palm follows the weight shift to rest opposite your inner right elbow. Your right arm is curved, guarding the groin. The upper part of your right arm faces forward.

Your feet remain at right angles to each other, unlike the other postures where the rear foot has come round to 45°.

LESSON 7
White Crane Spreads Wings.
Brush Left Knee and Push

1 Drop all your weight into your right leg. Turn your waist to the left. As your right hand begins to rise, your left hand sweeps down in front of your left thigh.

2 Pick up your empty left leg and touch the toe on the ground but without shifting your weight. Bring your right hand up to guard your temple, turning to face diagonally outwards as it moves up. Your left hand floats down, resting on a cushion of air outside the upper left leg.

3 As you turn your waist to the left, your right hand follows and sweeps down; your left palm opens outwards.

4 As you turn your waist to the right, your right hand continues in a circle. Your left hand follows the movement of your waist and faces palm down in front of your chest. As your waist returns to the centre, bring your right hand level with your shoulder, palm facing forwards.

5 Take a shoulder-width step with your left foot, heel first. Move 70% of your weight into your left leg as your left hand brushes down across it. Meanwhile, your right hand follows a con-cave curve into the centre to finish with the fingers in line with your mouth.

LESSON 8
Play Guitar. Brush Left Knee and Push
This posture is also known as "Strumming the Lute".

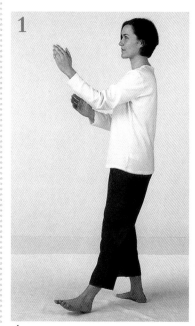

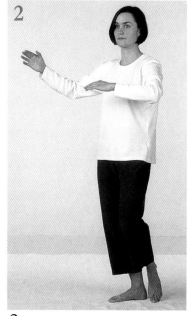

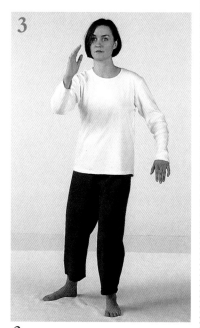

1 As all your weight sinks into your left leg, adjust the empty right foot by drawing it slightly nearer the left foot, toe first. Bring your weight into the right foot. Your left leg and arm float up simultaneously – imagine a thread connecting them – the left heel touching the ground but without weight. Ensure that the left leg would avoid contact with the right heel if drawn back.

2 Turn to the right, dropping your right hand down while your left hand follows the movement of your waist to the centre of your chest, palm facing down. As your waist returns to the front, your right hand comes to shoulder height, palm forwards.

3 Take a shoulder-width step with your left foot, heel first. Move 70% of your weight into your left leg as your left hand brushes down across it. Meanwhile, your right hand follows a concave curve into the centre to finish with the fingers in line with your mouth.

LESSON 9
Step Forward, Deflect Downwards, Intercept and Punch

1 Turn your waist 45° to the left and sink all your weight into your right foot. As your weight shifts back, lift the toes of your left foot and pivot 45° on the heel. Bring your hands down parallel with your left leg, just outside and in front of the thighs.

2 Shift all your weight into your left leg. Form a loose fist with your right hand as your body moves forward. Ensure that the fingers are not wrapped around the thumb. The right toes come up behind the left heel.

3 Arc both hands and your right foot simultaneously towards the centre line, as your waist turns to the right. The right foot lands empty, in line with the left instep.

4 Continue to turn your waist to the right, bringing the right fist palm upwards to rest on the right hip. Transfer all your weight to your right foot.

5 Place your left foot a shoulder width from the right foot. Shift 70% of your weight to your left leg and bring your right fist forward to punch, rotating it through a quarter turn in a corkscrew motion. Bring your left arm across your body, palm facing your inner right elbow.

LESSON 10
Withdraw and Push.
Crossing Hands

1 As you turn your waist to the left, your right arm follows your body to an angle of 45° and the fist opens up. Meanwhile, cup your left hand under your right elbow.

2 Draw your right arm across your left palm as your weight sinks into your right foot and your waist turns to the right.

3 Bring your waist back to the centre and turn both palms to face the front.

4 Move your weight forward 70% on to your left leg. Your hands remain at shoulder width and shoulder height.

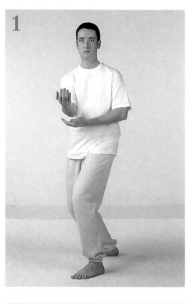

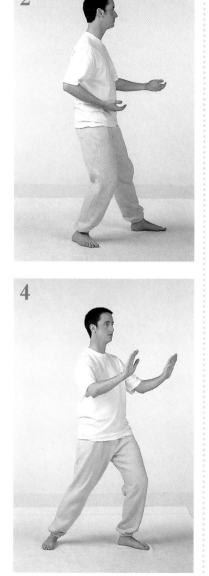

5 Turn your waist to the right and simultaneously sink all your weight into your left leg. Draw your hands in towards your chest in a softly inverted "V" shape, as if holding the top of a large ball.

6 As your whole weight shifts into your right leg, turn your waist to the right. Your left toes turn with your waist and your right hand travels out diagonally upwards.

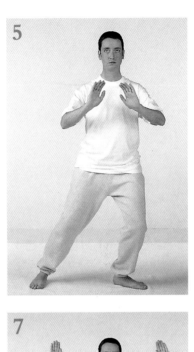

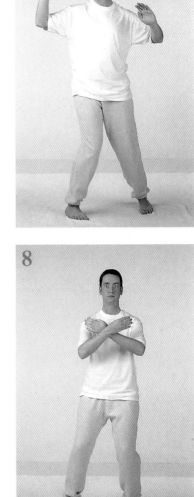

7 Sink all your weight back into your left leg. Your left hand now travels out diagonally.

8 Bring your right foot shoulder-width away from and parallel to the left, but maintain your weight 70% in the left leg. Both hands circle down and up, stopping opposite your chest, palms facing the body. The wrists are touching, with the right wrist outside the left one.

Lesson 11
Embrace Tiger, Return to Mountain

1 Keeping all your weight in your left leg, turn your waist to the right, pivoting on the ball of your right foot. Open your hands outwards. Step diagonally back with your right foot. Ensure the step is empty, and that the heels are shoulder-width apart. Move your weight 70% on to your right foot. As your waist completes its turn to the right diagonal, move your left hand so that the fingertips are in line with your left shoulder, palm facing forward. The right hand is palm up by the hip.

2 As you turn your waist slightly to the right, allow your left hand to come across so that the fingertips point to your right elbow. Meanwhile, your right hand travels upwards so that the fingertips point heavenward.

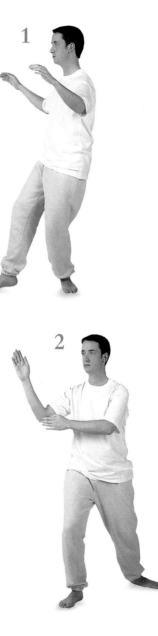

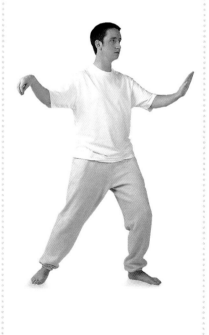

Lesson 12
Roll Back, Press and Push: Diagonal Single Whip

▼ Now repeat the sequence "Grasping the Sparrow's Tail" in Lessons 4 and 5. This time, perform this section from one diagonal corner to the other rather than from one side to the other. This picture shows your position at the end of the sequence, facing the corner.

LESSON 13
Punch under Elbow

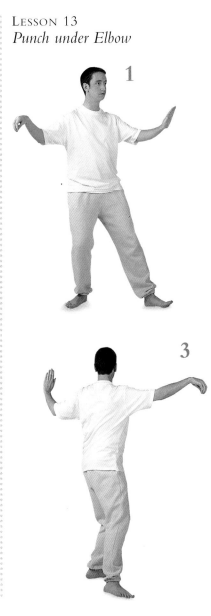

1 Sink all your weight back on to your right foot. Turn your waist 45° to the left, lifting the left toes and letting your left foot and both arms pivot 45° to the left.

2 Lower your left foot, gradually shifting weight forward into it. When all your weight is on your left foot, step forward with your right foot so that the heel is in line with your left instep.

3 Rotate your upper body 90° to the left. Your arms follow this waist movement, so that the hook (your right hand) is now out in front level with your right shoulder, and your left hand is level with your face at 90° to the front. Your weight is in your left leg.

4 Transfer all your weight to your right leg, turning your waist to the right and letting your left hand move down, then up, until the fingers are in line with your left shoulder. Your left arm and leg move around simultaneously. Rest your left heel on the ground without any weight. Meanwhile, turn your right hand into a loose fist and draw it towards your body to rest just inside your left elbow.

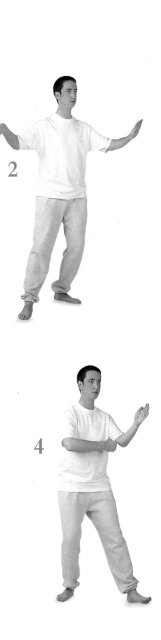

LESSON 14
Step Back to Repulse the Monkey: Right and Left

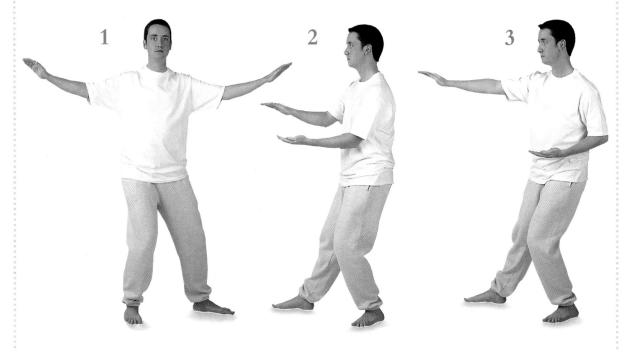

1 As you turn your waist further to the right, your right hand opens and moves down by your hip, then floats up to shoulder height. The palm of your left hand turns over to face down. Your eyes remain midway between your palms, with both hands staying in your peripheral vision.

2 Step back with your left foot as your waist turns to the left. Your right hand travels forward, palm facing down, while your left hand travels down towards your left hip with the palm facing upwards.

3 Feel the connection between the palms as your hands pass near each other. The right toes also straighten as the waist turns. As you continue to turn to the left, your left hand floats up to shoulder height, while your right hand comes forward, palm facing down, in a mirror image of Step 1.

LESSON 15
Step Back to Repulse the Monkey (Right).
Diagonal Flying

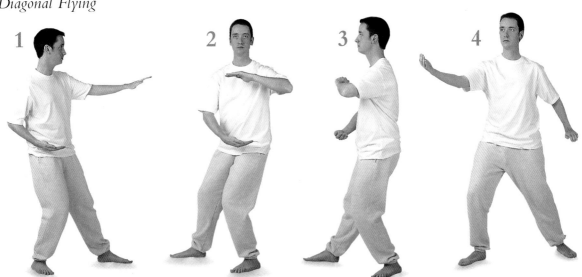

1 Turn your waist to the right, step back with your right foot and let your left hand travel forward, palm down. Your right hand moves down to rest on your hip, palm up. Your left foot turns to face the front as the waist moves. Your right hand now comes up to shoulder height, palm down, to return to the posture shown in Step 1 of Lesson 14 opposite.

2 With your weight on your left foot, turn your waist to the left. Turn your right hand palm upwards as it travels round in front of your waist, while your left hand, palm downwards, comes in front of your chest. Your hands are now holding an imaginary ball in front of your chest, with the left hand uppermost and the right hand directly below it.

3 Turn your waist 90° to the right, maintaining the position of your arms and hands in front of your chest, as if carrying the ball.

4 Stepping with your right foot, turn a further 135° to the right, and transfer 70% of your weight into the right foot. Your waist also turns to the right and your right hand moves with it, travelling to shoulder height, arm extended and facing diagonally upwards. Your left hand moves simultaneously to just outside your left thigh, palm facing down.

LESSON 16
Waving Hands in Clouds (Right, Left, Right)

1 Bring all your weight on to your right foot. Turn your waist to the right and move your left hand across near your right hip. At the same time, your right hand turns palm downwards at shoulder height. Raise your left foot and move it forward until the left heel is level with the right.

2 As your waist turns to the front, move your right hand to face it and your left hand to face your chest. The right toes swivel round to face forwards so that your feet are now shoulder-width apart.

3 As your waist turns to the left, turn your palms towards each other, as if holding a large ball to the left of your body. All your weight is in your left leg and your right foot steps in to half shoulder width.

4 Turn your waist back to the centre. Your hands again change position, the left hand descending to be opposite and facing your waist, and the right hand opposite and facing your chest.

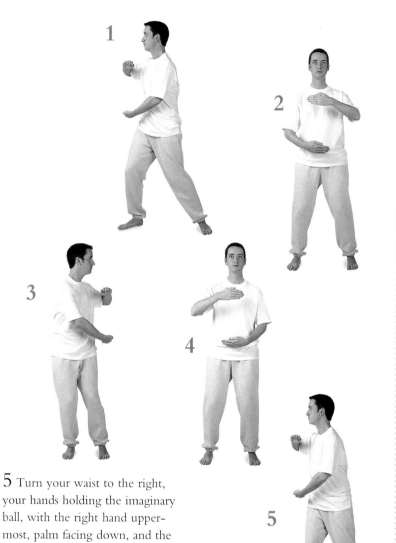

5 Turn your waist to the right, your hands holding the imaginary ball, with the right hand uppermost, palm facing down, and the left hand below it, palm facing up. When all your weight is on your right foot, step back to shoulder width with the left.

LESSON 17
*Waving Hands in Clouds (Left, Right, Left).
Single Whip*

1 Turn your waist back to the centre, bringing your right hand down to face your waist and your left hand up to face your chest. Repeat Steps 3, 4 and 5, then Steps 2 and 3 from Lesson 16.

2 Turn your waist back to the centre and form a hook with your right hand, as it moves in level with your chest, directly above your left hand which is located in front of your waist, palm upwards.

3 Step forward with your right foot. Turn your waist to the right, then to the left as you transfer your weight to your right foot, sending out the hook at 90° to the front of your body.

4 Continue turning your waist to the left and step with your left foot to shoulder width, with your left palm facing your left shoulder.

5 Shift your weight 70% on to your left foot, turning away your left palm at shoulder height, and turning the right toes to 45°.

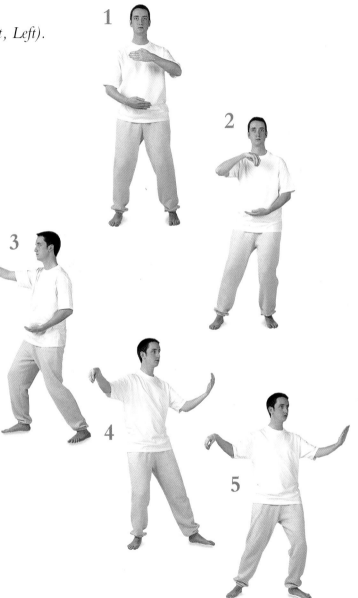

LESSON 18
Golden Rooster Stands on One Leg (Left). Squatting Single Whip

1 Sink all your weight into your left leg, turning your left hand over so that the palm faces upwards. Simultaneously turn out the right toes.

2 Move your weight across into your right leg, bringing your left palm in towards your chest. The left toes turn 45° to the right.

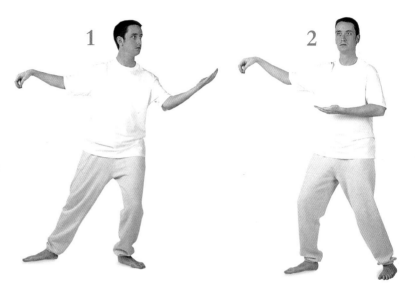

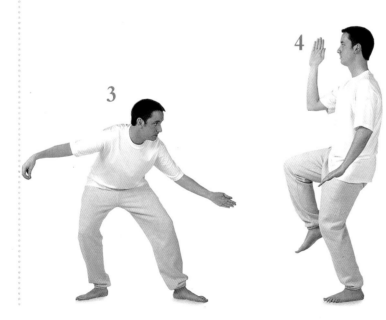

3 Sink down into your right leg, keeping your back straight. Move your waist to the left, brush open your left knee with your left arm and turn your left toes out 90° to the left.

4 Transfer all your weight into your left leg. Open the right hand hook, lower the hand then bring it up in front of your chest. Raise your right leg as your weight shifts forward into your left leg, so that your right thigh becomes parallel with the ground. Bend your left knee and let your left hand rest on a cushion of air by your left thigh.

LESSON 19
Golden Rooster Stands on One Leg (Right). Separate Right Foot

1 Place your right foot down and move all your weight on to it. As your weight sinks into your right leg, your right hand descends to rest on a cushion of air by your right thigh. Your left arm and left leg simultaneously move up to form a mirror image of the previous posture.

2 Step out with your empty left foot diagonally to the left, and form a ward-off position with your left arm horizontally across your body opposite your chest.

3 Shift all your weight into your left leg, bringing your right arm up to cross in front of your left arm, with the wrists touching. Bring your right toe to your left heel. Turn your wrists, maintaining skin contact as you do so, so that your left arm now crosses your right.

4 Then turn your hands away from your body, and open them out in a fan-like action.

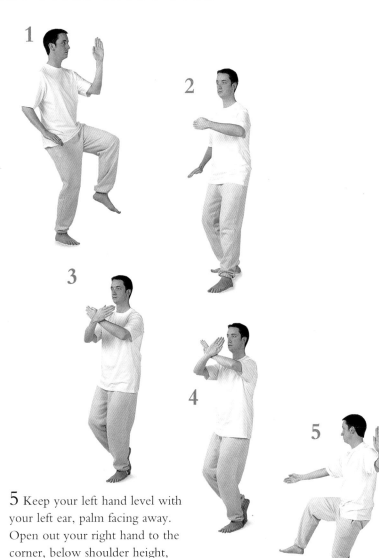

5 Keep your left hand level with your left ear, palm facing away. Open out your right hand to the corner, below shoulder height, and simultaneously kick gently with your right leg, to knee height.

LESSON 20
Separate Left Foot. Brush Left Knee and Push

1 Keeping all your weight in your left leg, turn to the left-hand corner, forming a ward-off position with your right arm.

2 Turn your waist to the right and step to the right with your right leg. As you transfer weight into it, bring your left hand up outside the right so that the wrists meet. The left toes come to the right heel.

3 Open out your hands, the right hand this time remaining level with the head and the left hand travelling to below shoulder height. The left foot follows, kicking gently to the corner.

4 Turn your waist and left knee to the front again. Take a shoulder-width empty step with your left leg, toes pointing forwards.

5 Brush your left hand across and above the front of your left leg, to just outside your left thigh. Your right hand curves in, fingertips forward, to finish with the fingers in line with your mouth.

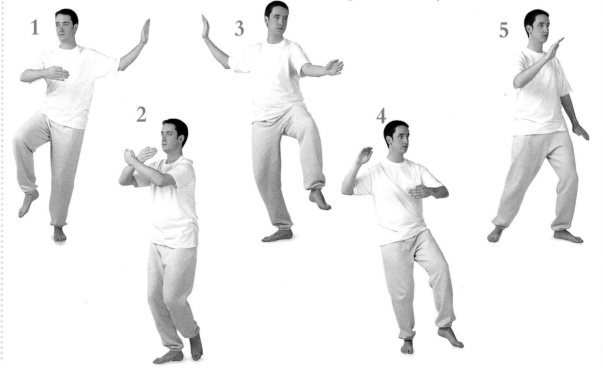

LESSON 21
Needles at Sea Bottom

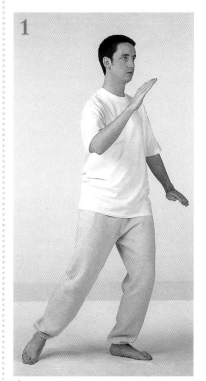

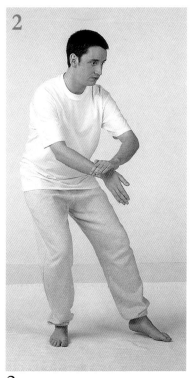

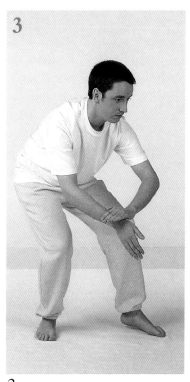

1 Move all your weight into your left leg. Pick up your empty right foot and make a small adjustment step forward.

2 Place your right toes down, then as you sink your weight into the foot, bring your left hand across your body so that the left palm rests above your right wrist. At the same time, pick up your left leg and place the toes down empty of any weight: all your weight is now in your right leg.

3 Move your right arm forwards and diagonally downwards with your body, then vertically downwards. The arm remains in line with your right leg, and all your weight remains in your right leg.

Lesson 22
Iron Fan Penetrates Back.
Turn Body, Chop and Push

1 As you raise your body, your weight remains in your right leg and both hands assume a ward-off position. Take a shoulder-width step with the left foot. Shift your weight 70% into your left leg and turn your hands outwards, the left hand in front of your mouth, the right hand guarding your temple.

2 Turn your waist to the right and sink all your weight back into your right leg, bringing your left toes round. Bring your left hand up, turning the palm diagonally outwards to guard the temple. At the same time, form a loose fist with your right hand, palm facing downwards in front of your chest.

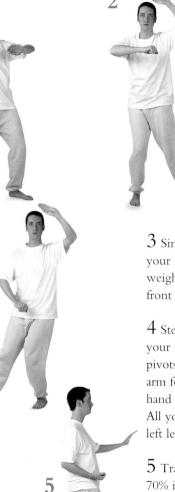

3 Sink all your weight back on to your left leg. As you transfer the weight back, the fist descends in front of your groin.

4 Step to shoulder width with your right foot. Your right arm pivots at the elbow and your left arm folds across so that the left hand faces the right inner elbow. All your weight remains on your left leg.

5 Transfer your weight forward 70% into your right leg. Your left arm pushes forward, fingertips in line with your left shoulder, and your right fist descends to your right hip, palm upwards. The left toes are at 45°.

LESSON 23
Step Forward, Deflect Downwards, Intercept and Punch, Kick with Heel

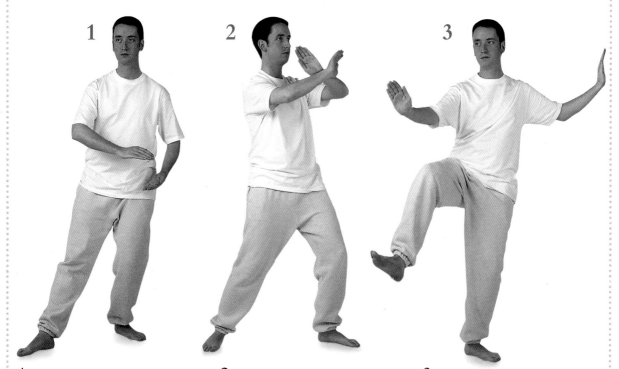

1 Sink all your weight back into your left leg as your waist turns to the left. Bring the right toe to the left heel. Your right hand comes across your body, the fist softens and the palm faces down by the left hip. The left hand is directly below the right hand, palm upwards. Now go back to Lesson 9 and repeat Steps 3, 4 and 5.

2 Sink your weight into your left leg, turning your waist to the right. Cross your wrists, the right outside the left. Sink your weight back into your right leg. Your waist turns left and your left foot pivots on the heel 45° to the left. Shift all your weight forward into your left leg, turning your hands palms outwards.

3 Open your hands out like a fan, the right hand to below shoulder height, the left hand at head height, palms facing away. Your right foot comes up from the ground and the heel kicks diagonally away.

LESSON 24
Brush Right Knee and Push. Brush Left Knee and Punch Down

1 Place your empty right foot on the ground, toes forward. Your right hand curves down to rest on a cushion of air outside your right thigh. Your left hand curves forward to push to the centre, fingertips in line with your mouth.

2 Sink back into your left leg, turning your waist to the right, the palm of your left hand facing your body in a ward-off position.

3 Transfer your weight forward into your right foot, with your left palm turning downwards.

4 When all your weight is in your right foot, take an empty shoulder-width step with your left foot, and bring 70% of your weight into it. Your right hand forms a loose fist, which comes up over your right hip and punches down into the centre. Your left hand brushes across your left leg and rests outside your left knee. Your back remains straight.

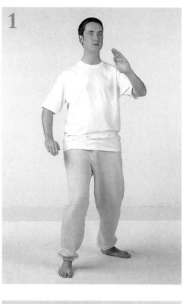

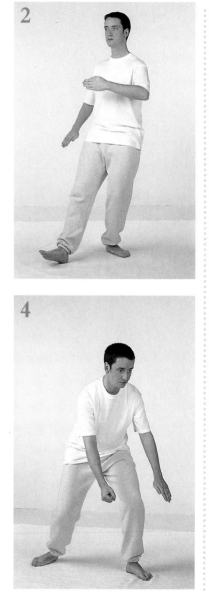

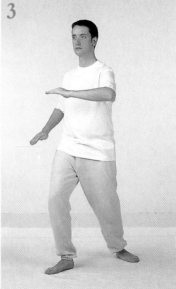

LESSON 25
Ward Off Right. Roll Back,
Press and Push. Single Whip

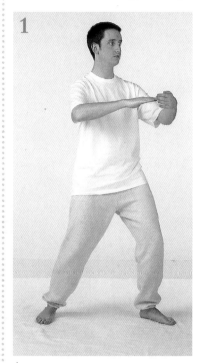

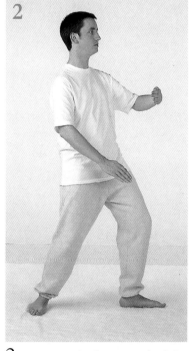

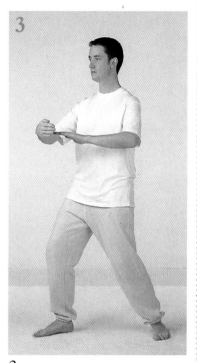

1 Sink back into your right leg. Your left hand assumes a ward-off position, the fingertips of your right hand pointing towards the centre of the left palm. Your right palm faces downwards.

2 Turn your body 45° to the left, pivoting on the left heel. Shift all your weight forward into your left leg. Your left arm remains in position, while your right hand presses down.

3 Step through at shoulder width with your empty right foot. As you transfer 70% of your weight into it, your right hand comes up into a ward-off position opposite your chest, with the left fingertips now pointing towards the right palm, left palm downwards. Now repeat Lessons 4 and 5.

LESSON 26
Fair Lady Weaves Shuttles (Right and Left)

1 Transfer your weight to your right leg as you turn your waist to the right, and turn the empty left toes through 90°. Bring your left hand across your body and under your elbow. Open the hook of your right hand and lower the right arm, palm turning upwards.

2 Sink your weight back into your left leg, turn your waist further to the right and turn out your right foot so the heel is in line with the left instep.

3 Sink your weight into your right leg, drawing your left arm across your right palm, and step at shoulder width to the left corner with your left foot. As you shift your weight forward into your left leg, turn both palms outwards, the left hand guarding your temple and the right in line with your mouth.

4 Transfer your weight into your right foot and turn your waist and left foot to the right as far as possible (135°). Turn your palms to face your body, the right palm by the left elbow.

5 Sink your weight back into your left leg and draw your left arm across your right palm.

6 Turn a further 135° right, to the corner. Step to shoulder width with your right foot, and shift 70% of your weight into it, pushing towards the centre of your mouth with your left hand. Bring your right hand up to guard your forehead, palm facing diagonally outwards.

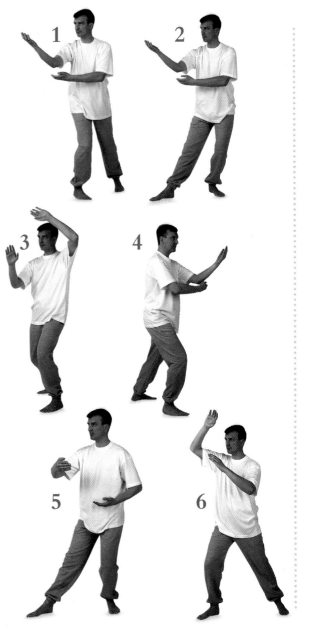

LESSON 27
*Fair Lady Weaves Shuttles
(Right and Left)*

1 Turn your waist 45° to the left, sinking all your weight into your left leg. Pick up your empty right foot and draw it inwards, toes pointing to the front. Transfer all your weight to your right foot, then step to the left corner (45°) with your left foot. Turn your palms in again and draw your right arm across the left palm, left arm remaining in a ward-off position.

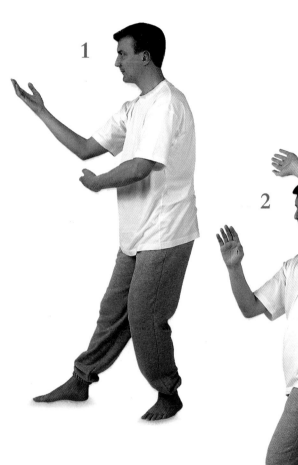

2 Your left hand then moves up and turns outwards by your head, while the fingers of your right hand come into the centre in line with your mouth. Now repeat the postures described in Steps 4, 5 and 6 of Lesson 26.

LESSON 28
Ward Off Left. Ward Off Right. Roll Back,
Press and Push. Single Whip

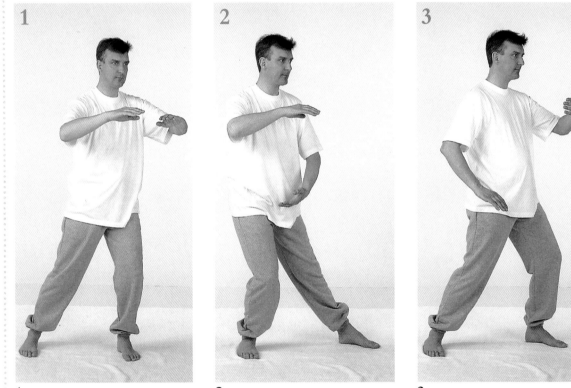

1 Sink your weight into your left leg as your waist turns to the left. Both arms come round with the movement of your waist, the left hand marginally lower than the right. The right toes come round to 45° from the front.

2 Sink your weight into your right leg as your left hand presses down, palm facing downwards. Take a shoulder-width step with your left foot.

3 Transfer your weight 70% into your left foot. Your left hand comes up in front of your chest, palm facing the body in a ward-off position. Your right hand floats on a cushion of air outside your right thigh. Now repeat the postures described in Lessons 3, 4 and 5.

LESSON 29
Squatting Single Whip, Step Forward to the
Seven Stars

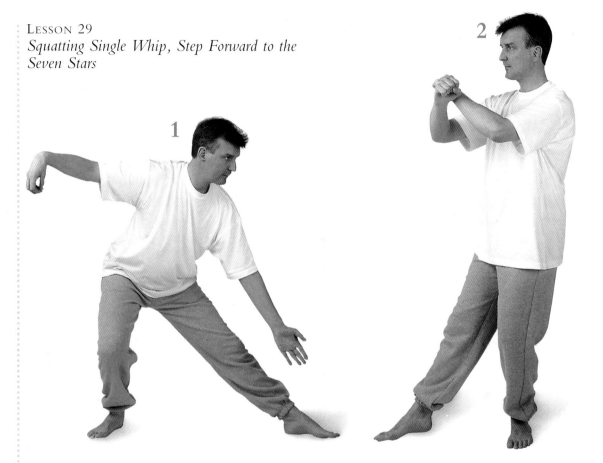

1 Repeat the postures described in Steps 1, 2 and 3 of Lesson 18, ending by brushing open the left knee.

2 Transfer all your weight into your left leg. The right hand hook opens and the hand descends, then comes up in front of your neck, where it forms a loose fist. At the same time, your left hand rises up to form a loose fist, and connects at the wrist inside your right hand. Move your right toes forward to touch the ground without weight.

LESSON 30
Step Back to Ride Tiger. Turn Body and Sweep Lotus with Leg

1 Keep your weight in your left leg and step back with your right foot, toes touching the ground first. Sink your weight into it and turn your waist to the right. The fists open and then move down by your right hip, wrists still connected.

2 Pick up your left leg as your waist turns right, then place your toes down as your waist turns back to the left. Your right hand comes around to the front with the movement of your waist, fingertips level with your right ear, and your left hand sweeps down across your body and left leg, to rest outside your left thigh.

3 Pick up your left toes, turn your waist to the left corner and place the toes down empty of any weight. Your right palm faces your inner left elbow. Your left hand is at the height of your left shoulder, elbow relaxed.

4 Lift your left toes and swing your waist clockwise, pivoting on the ball of your right foot. Your arms swing round to the right with the movement of your waist.

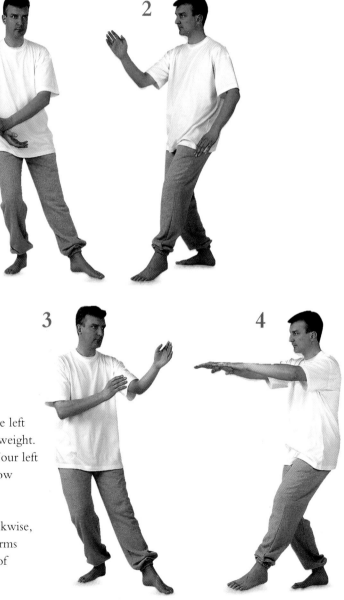

5 Drop your left foot and transfer all your weight into it straight away.

6 When your arms and waist reach the front (the arms at shoulder height and shoulder width with the palms facing downwards), your right foot lifts up and circles clockwise.

7 After circling, your right leg comes to rest with the upper leg parallel to the ground and foot relaxed. Your left leg is bent.

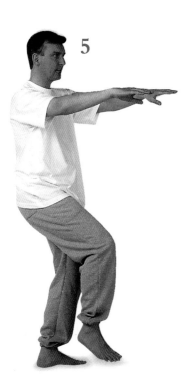

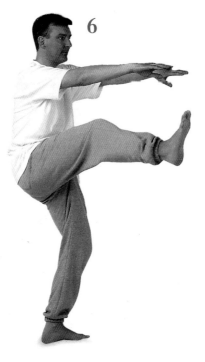

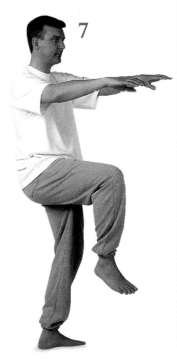

LESSON 31
*Bend Bow to Shoot Tiger.
Step Forward, Deflect
Downwards, Intercept and
Punch*

1 Turn your waist to the right.
Your arms follow your waist,
dropping down parallel, and your
right foot is placed facing the right
corner.

2 As your waist turns to the right,
shift your weight into your right
leg and circle your arms round to
the right of your waist. As your
waist turns back to the left, raise
your arms and circle round with
the waist movement. Form loose
fists with both hands. Bring the
right hand up to the right of your
forehead, knuckles facing your
right eyebrow. Your left hand
remains at shoulder height.
Continue turning your waist to
the left, keeping all your weight in
your right leg. Pick up your
empty left foot and make a small
adjustment step, the toe returning
to the ground first.

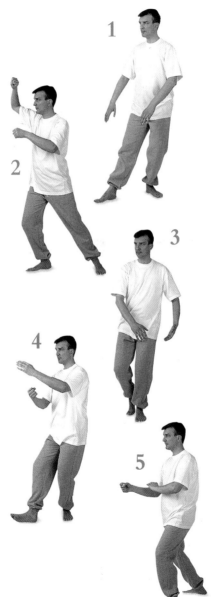

3 Sink your weight into your left
leg and pick up your right foot,
placing the toes by your left heel.
Open the left fist as your arms
move across your body following
the waist movement.

4 Both hands and your right foot
simultaneously arc towards the
centre line, as your waist turns to
the right. The right foot lands
empty, in line with the left instep.

5 Continue to turn your waist,
bringing the right fist palm
upwards to rest on your right hip
and shifting all your weight on to
your right foot. Step through at
shoulder width with your left foot.
Now shift 70% of your weight to
the left leg and bring your right
fist forward to punch, rotating
through a quarter turn in a
corkscrew motion. Your left arm
comes across your body, palm
facing your inner right elbow.

LESSON 32
Withdraw and Push. Crossing Hands. Conclusion, Attention

1 Repeat the postures described in Lesson 10. Ensure your weight is 70% in your left leg when crossing hands.

2 From crossing hands, turn both palms down to face the ground as your body rises up.

3 Bring all your weight into your left leg, turn your waist to the right and pivot on your left heel, turning the foot out to 45°.

4 Move all your weight into your right leg. Step in with your left foot so that the feet make a right angle with each other. Bring 50% of your weight back to the left foot. Rest your arms and hands naturally by the side of your body, with your shoulders relaxed. You are now ready to begin again!

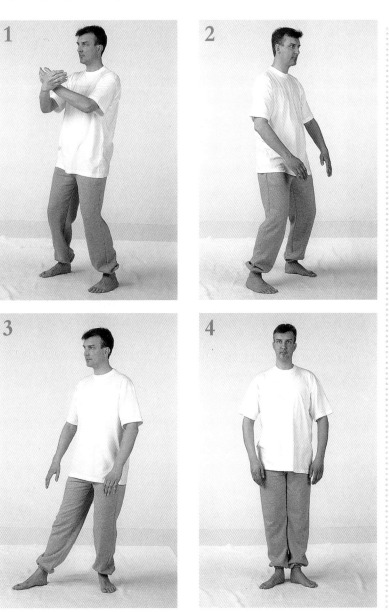

BIBLIOGRAPHY

Chinese Soft Exercise – A T'ai Chi Workbook, Paul Crompton, Unwin Paperbacks, 1986.

Movements of Magic: The Spirit of T'ai Chi Ch'uan, Bob Klein, Newcastle Publishing, 1984.

Tai Chi: Ten Minutes to Health, Chia Siew Pang & Goh Ewe Hock, Unwin Paperbacks, 1984.

There are no Secrets: Professor Cheng Man-ch'ing and his Tai Chi Chuan, Wolfe Lowenthal, North Atlantic Books, 1991.

The Way of Energy, Master Lam Kan Chuen, Gaia Books, 1991.

The Way of Harmony: A Guide to Soft Martial Arts, Howard Reid, Unwin Paperbacks, 1988.

PHOTOGRAPHY CREDITS

The majority of the pictures were taken by Don Last. The publisher would also like to thank Tony Stone Images p. 6 (Bob Thomason), p. 8 (Zigy Kaluzny); Zefa p. 2, p. 7; Jane Burton p. 11.

AUTHOR'S ACKNOWLEDGEMENTS

Sincere thanks to the many Tai Chi teachers who have encouraged and inspired me, including Peter Phipps, Pamela Hiley, Liz Fort, James Law, Osman Phillips, John Brewer, Peter Chin Kean Choy, Gerda Geddes, and Chung Liang Al Huang. To Arthur, Adriaan, Christian, Toby and Andy Winstanley for your enthusiasm, sharing and practice. To Bill Willis, Mick Sheridan, Jane Wolfson and Steve Rippl for your enthusiastic assistance in teaching. To Don and Penny for the photography (and tasty lunches), to models Mick, Esther, Steve and Ankin and to my editor Fiona. And finally, to dear Cheng Man-Ch'ing, whom I never had the good fortune to meet, my heartfelt thanks for bringing Tai Chi to the West, in a radical departure from tradition. You have brought me, and many thousands of others, much pleasure, confidence, health, awareness.... and relaxation!

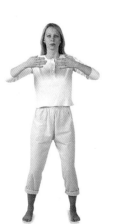
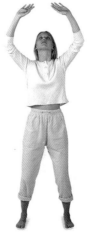
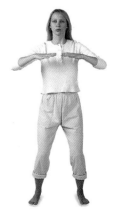